Published By:
Dennis Yang, M.Eng., L.Ac

This book is not intended to provide medical advice or to take the place of medical advice and treatment from your personal physician. Readers are advised to consult their own doctors or other qualified health professionals regarding the treatment of their medical problems. The author takes no responsibility for any possible consequences from any treatment, techniques, ideas, recommendations, opinions, advice, suggestions, action or application of medicine, supplement, herb or preparation to any person reading or following the information in this book. If readers are taking prescription medications, they should consult with their physicians and not take themselves off of medicines to start supplementation without the proper supervision of a physician.

Dennis Yang is a 2nd generation acupuncturist licensed by the Massachusetts Board of Registration in Medicine, specializing in orthopedic issues. He holds a Master of Acupuncture from the New England School of Acupuncture, and a B.S. and an M.Eng. in Electrical Engineering from the Massachusetts Institute of Technology.

To have Dennis Yang hold health seminars or speaking engagements you may contact:

Dennis Yang, M.Eng., L.Ac

63 Shore Road, Suite #11
Winchester, MA 01890
www.healingbyyang.com

Acknowledgements

I want to thank Lija, my wife, who encouraged me to leave the soul crushing high tech industry to pursue a lifelong dream of a career in healing, for her never ending love and support in all aspects of my life.

Introduction

This book is written for self-reliant contrarians like myself who will not accept the common misbelief that headaches can only be managed with medications, and take matters into, literally, their own hands to cure them. If you are willing to own your own health, this book is written for you.

An initial session for a new patient with headaches in my office typically goes something like this –

Me: "Please point at where you usually have a headache using one finger."
Patient: "I usually have a headache in the temple, forehead, and behind eyes in the morning and late afternoon" as tracing the headache regions with a finger.
Me: "Okay, are you having a headache right now?"
Patient: "No, not at the moment."
Me: "How about now?" as I squeeze a muscle in the front of the neck.
Patient: "Ah, yes, a headache is coming on right here" as pointing to the forehead.
Me: "Is this the same headache that you usually have?"
Patient: "Yes, it is."
Me: "How about now?" as I squeeze my fingers ½ inch higher along the same muscle.
Patient: "I feel it behind my eyes now."
Me: "In that case, I can probably create a headache in your temple if I do this" as I move my fingers even higher.
Patient: "Yes, you are."
Me: "Okay, I think I know what's causing your headache, and can cure it today."

If my patients tell me where they have their headaches, I can tell them where they come from. I am not talking about chemical or emotional origins of headaches here. I am talking about which muscles cause headaches where. Eliminating the headaches comes down to releasing the tension in the muscles that cause the headaches.

Most bodily pains behave like this, which is why knowing the precise location of the pain is the most important diagnostic factor in my practice. What is unique about headaches is that there is a near one-to-one mapping between the location of the headaches and the physical tissues that cause the headaches, whereas other pains usually have one-to-many mappings. This makes headaches much easier to treat, provided that the treatment techniques are performed correctly.

This book describes the treatment techniques in detail. I am a licensed acupuncturist, but the majority of my treatment techniques come from osteopathy. The techniques I present in this book are massage techniques that can be learned by non-medical professionals with a little bit of practice.

Chapter 1 – Causes of Headaches

Widespread Incomplete Theories

Vascular Dilation or Constriction

Once popular for explaining migraine headaches was the theory that vasodilation in the cranial blood vessels caused them.[1] This is true to a large degree, which is why Imitrex (vasoconstrictor medicine) works wonders for some migraine headache sufferers.[2] However, subsequent research results have shown that it is sometimes vasoconstriction that causes the migraine headaches, sometimes both vasodilation and vasoconstriction, or sometimes neither of them, which is why Imitrex does not work for other migraine headache sufferers.[3]

From a mechanical point of view, if the blood flows from left to right in a blood vessel and there is a pinch somewhere in the blood vessel, the blood vessel to the left of the pinch will dilate due to increased blood pressure, and the blood vessel to the right of the pinch will constrict due to decreased blood pressure. What will fix the coexistence of vasodilation and vasoconstriction is not to systemically vasoconstrict, which will further constrict the right side, or vasodilate, which will further dilate the left side, but to remove the pinch. This pinch is caused by abnormal tension in muscles that cross the blood vessel. Technically, it can be other soft tissues other than muscles, such as tendons, ligaments, nerves, fascia, etc., but since releasing the tension in the muscles results in releasing these soft tissues as well, I will collectively call them muscles in the rest of the book for practicality and brevity.

To illustrate my point, I once had a patient who would instantly get a supraorbital headache whenever he drank more than a sip of beer. Alcohol is a vasodilator at low levels, and vasoconstrictor at high levels, so it is tricky to treat alcohol induced headaches with either vasodilator or vasoconstrictor.[4] Upon examination, his right sternocleidomastoid muscle had a knot that, when squeezed, would create the exact same headache. He was very excited to go home and drink a whole can of beer without having a headache after one treatment.

Nerve Entrapment

Nerve entrapment theory explains headaches in a much more straightforward manner than vascular dilation or constriction theory. When a sensory nerve is irritated, the brain interprets it as pain, and a headache is simply nerve pain in the head.[5,6] The irritation typically occurs at places where the nerve curves abruptly, penetrates through a small foramen, or is compressed by a tight muscle.[7] These places are called entrapment sites. For example, the supraorbital nerve is often entrapped at the supraorbital foramen, causing frontal headaches during menstruation.[8]

My clinical observation validates this theory. The problem, however, is that this theory is not applied correctly in the medical field. The treatment protocol, based on nerve entrapment theory, is to inject a nerve blocking agent at the entrapment sites. With the supraorbital nerve entrapment example, for instance, the nerve blocking agent is injected at the layers of muscles that cover the supraorbital foramen, such as frontalis, to prevent the muscles from contracting, hence eliminating the irritation to the supraorbital nerve. This protocol will work, but only until the nerve blocking agent wears out. A more permanent solution is eliminating what causes the tension in the frontalis to begin with.

A muscle often stays contracted because the communication between the brain and the muscle is interrupted. Re-establishing the interrupted communication rapidly releases the contraction, usually within seconds. Continuing with the supraorbital nerve entrapment example, the frontalis is innervated by the facial nerve.[9] When the supraorbital nerve is pinched by the frontalis, the facial nerve is often entrapped by the sternocleidomastoid muscle near the styloid process. Therefore, releasing the tension in the sternocleidomastoid muscle near the styloid process will free the facial nerve entrapment, which will re-establish the interrupted communication from the brain to the frontalis. Once this communication is re-established, the frontalis releases its contraction within seconds, no longer pinching the supraorbital nerve, and the frontal headache disappears. In my opinion, this is how the sternocleidomastoid muscle is often responsible for frontal headaches.

Patients with chronic headaches come to my office often after multiple sessions of nerve blocking injections have failed them. The injection sites usually consist of sensory nerve entrapment sites and nerve roots at the cervical spine. It is no wonder that these treatments failed. Nerve entrapment theory would have helped a great number of headache sufferers if muscle relaxants were injected into the muscles that pinched the motor nerves of the muscles that entrapped the sensory nerves, rather than nerve blockers at the sensory nerve entrapment sites. For this reason, the currently practiced protocol of this model does not produce long term effects.

Muscle Tension

Popular among manual therapists is the theory that tension in the muscles or fascia lines causes headaches by pulling on parts of the head aberrantly. I too, find this theory to be valid. Trapezius and levator scapula cause occipital headaches by, directly and constantly, pulling on their attachments to the skull, for example.

This theory, however, falls short in explaining headaches in the vertex, frontal, retro-orbital, and temporal regions. Massaging muscles in these regions do not alleviate headaches as these headaches are caused by tension muscles that are a distance away and do not seemingly have a direct connection to these regions. This is where the trigger point theory comes into play.

Trigger Point

Recently popularized by the dry needling of orthopedic acupuncturists and physical therapists, Janet Travell's trigger point theory is about specific muscle knots that refer pain either onto itself or tissues some distance away.[10] When these muscles knots are treated with acupuncture needles or massage, a release takes place signified by a local twitch response, and the disappearance of the referred pain results.[11] This theory works the best for alleviating headaches among the theories discussed thus far.

Despite its tremendous effectiveness, there is a heated debate as to whether the referral pain is indeed caused by muscle knots themselves, or the muscle knots are simply entrapping peripheral nerves. This is because the referral pain patterns do not follow known physiological tissue trajectories; neither myofascial lines nor peripheral nerve distributions adequately explain the referral pain patterns.

While working amazingly well for many orthopedic cases, the current practice of trigger point therapy focuses on releasing individual muscles at most, and primary/satellite trigger points at best. Further development on the application of trigger points is desired. More specifically, the chain of hierarchy in muscles and muscle groups in terms of biomechanics and nerve innervations is necessary to determine the correct order of muscle releases. I make an attempt to provide this chain or hierarchy in this book.

Others

There are other theories that try to explain the causes of headaches. The organ and channel theories from Eastern medicine, food allergies, barometric pressure, and emotional stress are some of the widely known theories. Just like the theories explored previously, they are all correct to a degree. I will not explore them in any depth for two reasons. One, rather than discussing them in detail, and pointing out the shortcomings of them, I would rather start talking about what my theory is. Readers will have noticed that my approach to remedy the shortcomings of the theories discussed thus far comes down to finding and releasing tension in the correct muscles in the correct order. Two, these theories do not have much to do with my theory, and therefore, discussion on them will not help the reader understand my theory unlike the four theories that were covered in depth.

My Current Working Theory

Before discussing my theory, I feel that it is important for the readers to know a little bit about my background to understand how my theory came to life.

My father was an acupuncturist in South Korea, and I grew up assisting him since I was in kindergarten. Acupuncture needles, suction cups, moxa, magnets, etc. were some of my toys growing up. I have studied over a dozen acupuncture styles and other Eastern healing modalities along with Western osteopathy over the past 40 or so years since then. Needless to say, I am very acutely aware of what the Eastern medicine can and cannot do. I have no delusions about the clinical efficacy as well as limitations of Eastern medicine. I am also very aware of the historical propaganda of Taoism being the basis of the Eastern medicine and the myths of the ancient wisdom.

I received my undergraduate and graduate degrees in Electrical Engineering from the Massachusetts Institute of Technology. I have enough science background to understand the research and clinical application of the Western medicine, not to mention the political and economical influences that have been put upon it. Having lost my mother to the "miracle" of modern Western medicine, rather than to the diseases that plagued her, I am painfully aware of the chasm between the researchers and the clinicians. In short, I have learned not to blindly believe what the ancient or modern, the East or West has to say.

What I do believe, however, is the clinical results. No matter how brilliant or authoritative a theory is, if it does not produce results in the clinic, then it is useless. A theory should not dictate what and how a treatment is to be rendered to a patient even if it seemingly explains the mysteries of the universe. A human body is more complex than a theory. Instead, a theory should be derived from clinical observation to attempt to explain what is observed. A patient deserves more than academic musings, professional homage, cultural pride, and economic interests.

My way of honoring my patients is, and has always been, to do that which works. Although I am licensed in acupuncture, I rarely use acupuncture needles unless I know it is the best treatment tool. If a patient has breathing difficulty, I would release the diaphragm and the phrenic nerve (a nerve that innervates the diaphragm), with my hands, rather than needling some lung acupuncture points because the manual technique is incomparably more effective than acupuncture in this case. On the other hand, if a patient has numbness in the dorsum of the foot, I would needle the peroneus longus to release the entrapment of the peroneal nerve (a nerve that innervates the top of the foot), rather than applying fancy osteopathic nerve manipulation techniques, because acupuncture would resolve the problem incomparably faster than any other manual techniques that I know of. I am not married to any one way of healing.

My theory on the causes of headaches has emerged from applying different techniques from numerous schools of thought, retaining what worked and throwing away what did not. It was formed as an explanation for what I had witnessed through this process.

Keep in mind that the theory and techniques I am presenting in this book reflects my current understanding. As I evolve as a healer, the theory will evolve as well. The theory presented in this book is the latest snap shot in its evolution.

From successfully treating so many patients who did not get relief from headache clinics and other modalities, I slowly became aware that my approach was rather unique and truly effective. Medical doctors typically sought to alleviate headaches with medications, which aimed to either vasoconstrict or vasodilate. Neurologists injected nerve blockers near the entrapment sites of irritated sensory nerves. Manual workers focused on massaging the posterior muscles of the neck, typically forgetting the anterior muscles of the neck or on the face. They all worked, and they all failed. Perhaps the approach I was taking was combining all these approaches while filling in the missing components although I was not aware it at that time.

My approach is simply this; release tensions in the muscles (1) that are pinching the blood vessels so that there is no vasodilation or vasoconstriction, (2) that are pinching the motor nerves that innervate the muscles that pinch the sensory nerves, (3) that are directly pulling on the tissues in the head, (4) and that create referral pain in the head in the order that is neurologically and biomechanically correct.

When these tight muscles are released, the relief of the headache is immediate, hence curing the headache within an hour-long session in most cases. The clinical data I have gathered over the years support the theory that the tension is in 6 muscles; sternocleidomastoid, temporalis, scalene, trapezius, levator scapula, and masseter. The only diagnostic factor that is needed to figure out which muscle or muscles cause the headache is the locations of the headaches. This is because there is near a one-to-one mapping between the location of the headaches and muscles that cause the headaches.

What I mean by the word "mapping" is this; as long as the patients tell me accurately where the pain is, I can tell them which muscle the headache comes from. To achieve accuracy, I always ask them to use one finger to locate and trace where the headache is. To confirm this map, I squeeze the source of the headache to turn the headache on, and let go of the muscle to turn the headache off. Yes, I can turn the headache on and off by irritating a specific part of the muscle to demonstrate to my patient that the irritated part of the muscle is what causes the headache. What this means is that the causes of the headaches are mechanical, not chemical. This book is about the map that tells you which muscle tension causes headaches where, and how to dissolve the tension so that the associated headache disappears.

The chemical causes, however, still play a role in that they help the muscle tension to persist. When chemical intervention, in the form of medication or diet changes, takes place, it can help this perpetuating effect disappear, but more often than not, the muscle tension stays until it is mechanically dissolved.

My current theory is not without shortcomings. It does not address more complicated causes, which require professional care. A few examples are listed below.

- Maxilla deviation causing sinus issues – releasing the tension in the masseter is usually sufficient for acute sinus problems, but maxilla deviation usually needs to be corrected for chronic sinus problems. This is done through a sophisticated osteopathic technique

- Tumor in the brain – the tumor is simply taking up space, squeezing the surrounding tissues. A surgical intervention is needed
- Chemical triggers – wheat, alcohol, aspartame, MSG, etc. are some of the well-known headache triggers. The diet needs to be cleaned up. Note that there is a big difference between causes and triggers. Causes are the fundamental reasons for headaches, e.g., tension in the 6 muscles listed above. As such, without the causes, triggers do not induce a headache. My patient whose headache was triggered by alcohol prior to sternocleidomastoid muscle release is an example of this.

Following my approach will not cure headache examples like above. However, temporary relief will typically be seen lasting several days to a few months.

Chapter 2 – Map of Headaches

The presentation based classification of headaches, e.g., tension headache, migraine headache, cluster headache, sinus headache, rebound headache, etc. is used in allopathic medicine, but is meaningless as the same set of medications is used regardless of the classification.

The location based classification of headaches, on the other hand, points to where the headaches come from because there is a near one-to-one mapping between the location of the headaches and physical tissues that cause the headaches. The mapping I have discovered over time is depicted in the following pictures.

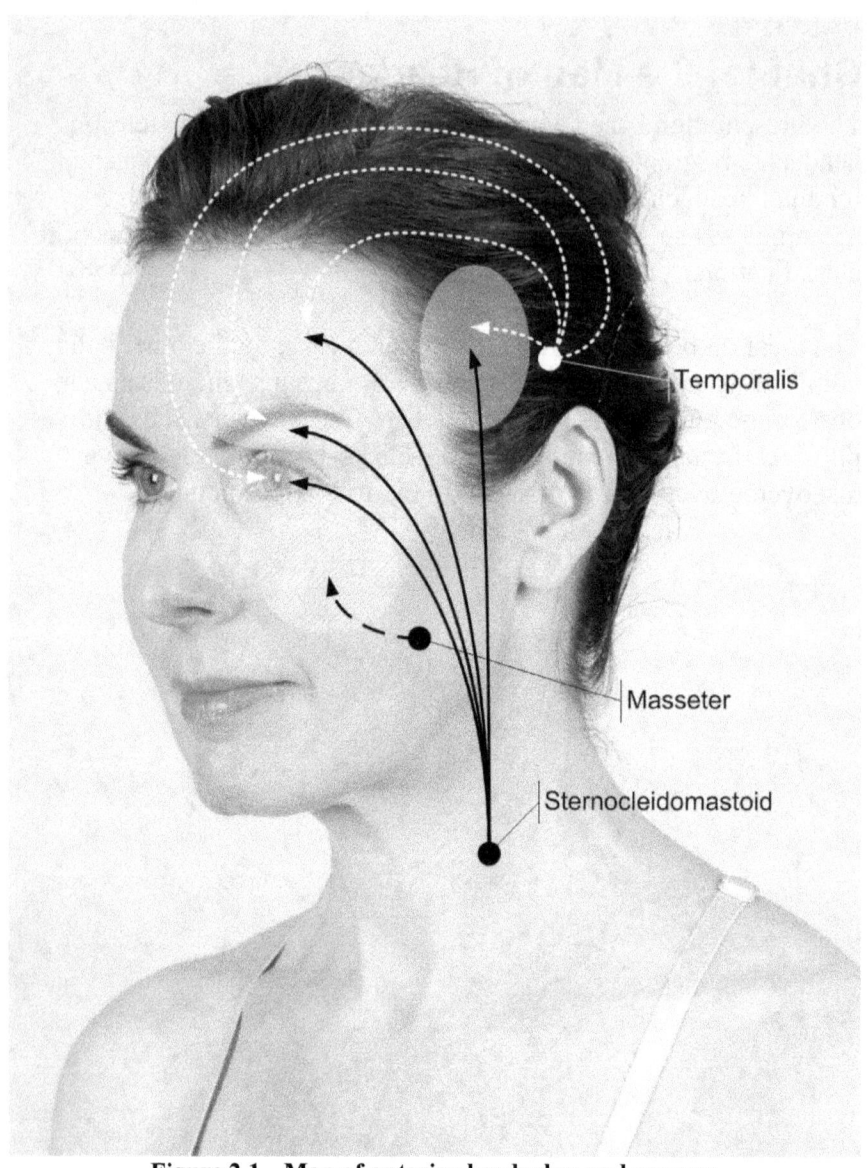

Temporalis

Masseter

Sternocleidomastoid

Figure 2.1 - Map of anterior headaches and sources

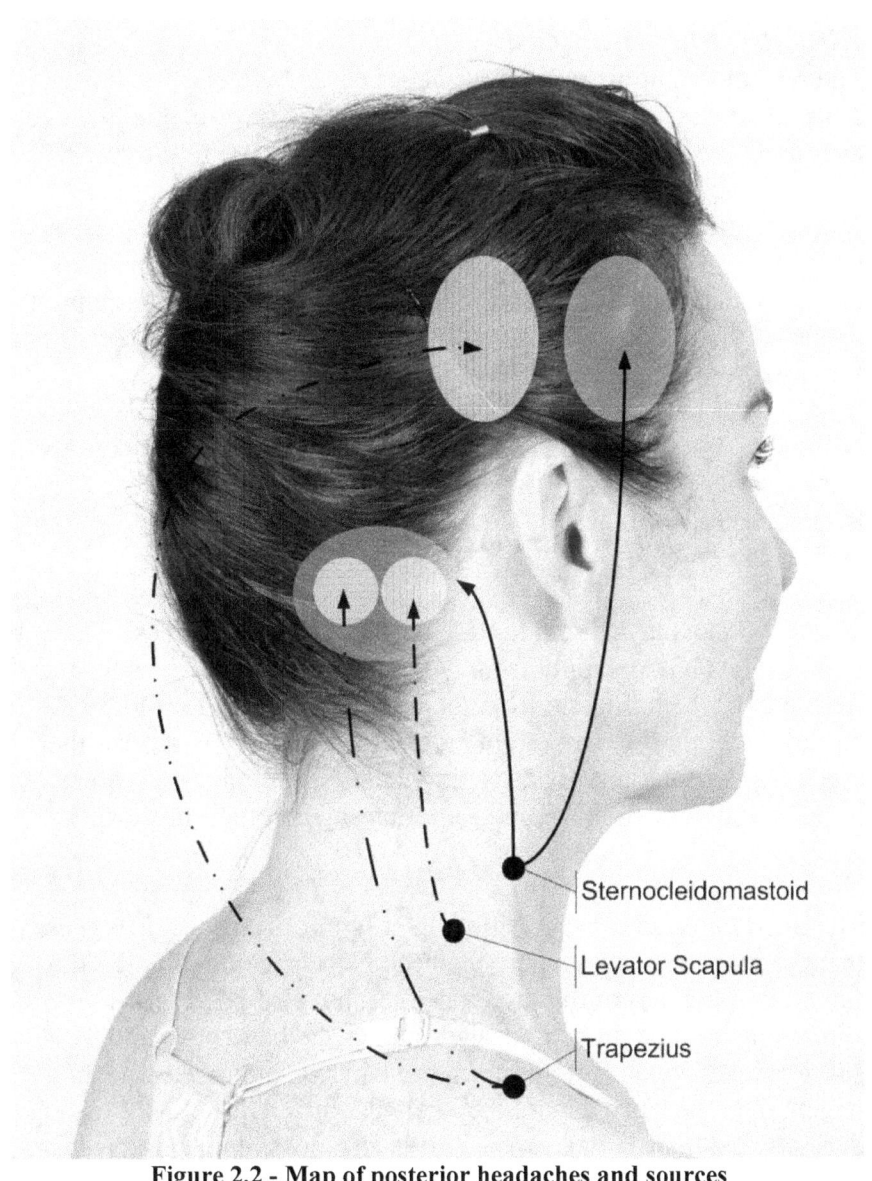

Figure 2.2 - Map of posterior headaches and sources

Sternocleidomastoid

The typical locations of the headaches caused by the sternocleidomastoid (SCM) are the frontal, above or behind the eyes, temporal, and occipital areas.[12] Most headaches are felt in one or more of these areas. I have found that nearly all headaches are caused by the SCM, or have it as the main cause of the headaches while a few other muscles play a support role. The prevalence of this is so high that if the location of the headache is hard to pinpoint, releasing the SCM will most likely resolve the headache at least for a few weeks, if not months.

Different parts of the SCM cause a headache in different locations.[13] It is as if these different parts are different muscles altogether. This is most likely from the fact that different parts of the muscle entrap different nerves.

The SCM also plays a role in vascular causes of headaches. The brain gets its blood supply from the internal carotid arteries for the front part of the brain and from the vertebral arteries for the back part of the brain.[14] The bottom part of the SCM can compress the common carotid artery, constricting the blood supply to the anterior brain. Patients with this condition often say that their heads feel foggy.

The SCM can also cause positional vertigo or dizziness. My guess is that the brain perceives where the head is in space not only by the function of the labyrinth in the inner ear, but also by the relative shortening and lengthening of the SCM as the head moves in the space. If the signals coming from the labyrinth and the SCM do not match, then the brain cannot reconcile the difference quickly enough during which vertigo takes place. It is also possible that the fascia connection of the SCM to the inner ear may interfere with the proper function of the labyrinth. Again, these are my guesses, not researched facts. But, I have cured too many positional vertigo cases by releasing the SCM not to mention it.

I have found that the right SCM is almost always the main culprit, regardless of which hand is the dominant hand, or which shoulder is higher than the other. On most patients even without headaches, the right SCM is bigger and tenser than the left. I have seen only two patients whose left SCM was bigger and tenser in all of my years of practice. A group of Japanese acupuncturists believe that when the right SCM is tenser, the patient is sympathetic dominant, and when the left side is tenser, parasympathetic dominant, but I do not find this to be true. This phenomenon remains a mystery to me. My guess is that the larger lobe of the liver is on the right side, pulling the right shoulder down more than the left side, so the SCM on the right side constantly has more load than the left, making it bigger and tighter. When I work on the ribs on my patients, the right side is almost always more rigid than the left.

Patients with this muscle pathology often sleep on one side, making one side shorter than the other, or on their stomach, which really makes one side shorter than the other, or sleep on the back using multiple pillows or down pillows that tilt the head forward excessively.

Temporalis
The headache locations caused by temporalis are eerily similar to those caused by the SCM. While temporalis and the SCM can independently create headaches, they often work together to create headaches. More specifically, the SCM creates a headache first, and if this headache is located in the temporalis, the temporalis starts to perpetuate the headache.[15] For this reason, the SCM and the temporalis should always be treated together, first the SCM followed by the temporalis.

The distinguishing characteristic with headaches stemming from the temporalis is that cold temperature, wind, or cold wind triggers the headache, and is often unbearable enough to make you cry.[16] I have seen patients who experienced headaches whenever driving with the window open in chilly weather, and a patient whose headache would get triggered by the cold air from an air conditioner.

Patients with the temporalis tension often grind their teeth at night, have jaw pain, or the upper and lower teeth are not aligned properly. They also tend to be side sleepers.

Levator Scapula

Levator scapula, along with the trapezius, causes occipital headaches. When the levator scapula is the primary cause, rotation of the head is very restricted. Instead of rotating the head, the patient will rotate the torso, or turn the eyes instead.[17] The difficulty with the rotation does not happen when the trapezius is the primary cause.

Patients with the levator scapula tension will also experience stiffness in the neck along the muscle from the posterolateral aspect of the neck toward the superior angle of the scapula when turning the head to the other side.[18] This stiffness is usually the chief complaint, rather than the headache in many cases. The trajectory of the trapezius tension is slightly different. It goes from the nape of the neck toward the shoulder (acromion process).

Despite the differences between the levator scapula and trapezius, they need to be treated together just like the SCM and temporalis pair. This is because they are synergists, serving the same mechanics in a variety of movements. What this means is that when one muscle is chronically tired, the other muscle needs to work harder to compensate to a point where an injury occurs.

Trapezius

Trapezius, along with the levator scapula, causes occipital headaches.[19] It can also cause temporal headaches, but is a minor contributor compared with the SCM and temporalis pair.

This is a favorite muscle for massage therapists for a good reason; it is a huge muscle where lots of stress tends to settle. However, massaging this muscle alone often fails to produce lasting results. This is because the tension in this muscle is often a result of spinal accessory nerve entrapment by the scalenes.[20] The spinal accessory nerve is what innervates the trapezius, and arises from the C1-C6 spinal nerve roots.[21] The three heads of the scalenes are attached to the transverse processes of C1-C7 and to the 1st and the 2nd ribs.[22] When the scalenes are shortened, the intervertebral foramen through which the cervical nerve roots come out of the vertebrae become narrow, and can entrap the nerves. Without releasing the shortened scalenes, the trapezius will not let go of its tension. The scalenes need to be treated before the levator scapula and the trapezius get their turn.

The scalenes also play a role in vascular causes of headaches. The brain gets its blood supply from the internal carotid arteries for the front part of the brain and from the vertebral arteries for the back part of the brain.[23] The vertebral arteries go through the transverse foramen of the cervical vertebrae. Shortened scalenes can compress the tissues surrounding the transverse foramen, thereby constricting the blood supply to the posterior brain. Patients with this condition often say that their heads feel foggy.

Masseter

The masseter is a very interesting muscle. For a long time, I attributed sinus congestion and pressure to an immune system response to things like the common cold. What I have found, quite accidentally, is that whether it is the congestion or pressure, the sinus issue is often caused by tension in the masseter.

Even if the sinus issue comes from catching the common cold, much of it, or almost all of it, can disappear when the masseter of the same side is thoroughly released if you treat it early enough or if it lingers long after all the other cold symptoms have disappeared. This muscle can easily be self-massaged, so next time you have a sinus problem, give it a try.

There are two layers in the masseter; one goes deep towards the ear from the mandible, and the other shallow one goes to the cheek bone. The layer that causes the sinus headache is the shallow one that goes to the cheek bone.[24]

Just like with the temporalis, patients with masseter tension often grind their teeth at night, have jaw pain, or the upper and lower teeth are not aligned properly. In this case, the pterygoid muscles need to be released as well, but that is beyond the scope of this book as the external pterygoid muscle can only be released with a long instrument such as an acupuncture needle longer than 40mm, and the internal pterygoid muscles can only be released intraorally.

Patients will oftentimes experience that one side of the face is affected more than the other. Typically, the side that is more affected has the jaw moved away from it toward the other side. I suspect that this puts more strain on the affected side by constantly pulling it. This jaw deviation can be fixed with osteopathic techniques, but that is beyond the scope of this book.

Chapter 3 – Fasciculation

To reiterate, headaches largely come from muscle tension itself, referral pain that the muscle tension creates, nerves that the muscle tension pinches, and the blood vessels that the muscle tension constricts, and releasing the muscle tension makes the headaches disappear.

Some readers may find the statement above too simplistic, or even wrong. What about joint misalignment that creates the muscle tension? How about the neural buds that interfere with the nerve impulses? You forgot about the hormones and chemicals in our food that can cause swelling of the nerves in the perforating canal or calcification of the canal itself?

What I have clinically witnessed is that the only set of techniques that consistently worked again and again is releasing the muscle tension with a cure rate of greater than 50% of acute or chronic headaches of any type, frequency, intensity, and location with one treatment session, and greater than 95% with 2 – 4 treatment sessions. Therefore, while the other causes may contribute to headaches, the contribution seems quite minor.

The remaining 5% or so of patients have complex causes that require advanced osteopathic techniques, and writing about them would turn this book into something for professional healers, and not for patients themselves. Also, note that if the perpetuating factors exist, they need to be treated in order to have a permanent cure, but that is also beyond the scope of this book. However, even with the perpetuating factors present, headaches, when treated properly as presented in this book, will go away for at least a few months, which is a much-needed break some readers would dream of.

The biggest challenge of writing this book has been how to let the readers know whether they are doing the massage techniques properly or not. What is the secret ingredient that turns regular massage to a miracle that can cure decades old headaches in one session? It is something called "fasciculation" also known as a local twitch response.

Fasciculation is the single most distinguishing characteristic of my healing regardless of whether I use acupuncture, tuina, or osteopathy. Basically, when my techniques have been applied correctly, fasciculation takes place in the tissues that the techniques have been applied to. This "jerking" of the tissues is perceptible not only to the healer, but to the patient as well although the degree of the perceptibility depends on the sensitivity of the individual. When the fasciculation stops in one area, all the healing that the local tissues can handle for that session is completed, and it is time to move onto the next area. Fasciculation is how the readers can be sure that the techniques have been applied correctly and healing has taken place.

When I first encountered this concept, it was from reading Janet Travell's book called *Myofascial Pain and Dysfunction*. She describes it as "a transient contraction of essentially those muscle fibers in the tense band."[25] She further elaborates "only if they harbor active trigger points."[26] This idea served me well for a couple of years in the beginning of my career. Over time, however, I have developed a different view point on the term because I have noticed that I was actually fasciculating not only the muscles, but also tendons, ligaments, nerves, blood vessels, and even internal organs.

The importance of fasciculation cannot be overemphasized. If fasciculation takes place, immediate pain relief follows. If there is no fasciculation, no healing has taken place, at least in my practice. I fasciculate regardless of the healing modalities and techniques I use in all the tissues I treat. All the advanced manual training I have received comes down to fasciculation.

To induce fasciculation, the usual stroking or kneading type of massage techniques need to be replaced with steady pressure. The amount of pressure cannot be too light like typical cranial therapy touch; the tissues have no reasons to respond. Nor can it be too heavy like Rolfing; the tissues will contract further to protect themselves. The pressure needs to meet the pressure the tissues exert back. It takes some time to learn just how much pressure to exert, but once one fasciculation is experienced, play with varying amount, angle, and order of the tissues treated, etc., to induce bigger and more frequent fasciculation. The treatment is complete when the fasciculation stops at each part of the tissues that you are treating.

Just like fingerprints, different individuals have a wide range of responses to massage in terms of fasciculation. People younger than early twenties typically respond very easily with large twitches. People who do not hold emotional stress, regardless of age, respond just as well. People who have taken any sort of pain medication within the past 48 hours are hard to get a response from. People who have chronically taken pain medication, especially recreational drugs can be nearly impossible. I have not found any differences between genders.

Chapter 4 – Techniques

The most difficult part of writing this book was about how to verbally describe my techniques, which primarily consist of orthopedic acupuncture needling and sophisticated osteopathic techniques, into methods that can be done by a lay person. This chapter is my best effort in doing exactly that. A video of these techniques will follow at a later date.

Once you find the area that matches with the location of your headache from the map of headaches, find the muscles that cause the headache, and release the tension in them following the techniques presented in this chapter. Keep in mind that the SCM and the temporalis act as if they are one muscle as far as headaches are concerned, therefore, they both need to be treated together, the SCM followed by the temporalis. Also, keep in mind that the scalenes need to be treated prior to treating either levator scapula or trapezius. The masseter can be treated all by itself.

Make sure that your fingernails are cut short and well filed before attempting any of the techniques to avoid not only injuring the skin, but also making the patients tense up from the unnecessary pain caused by sharp or long nails. I am illustrating the manipulation techniques on the right side of the body only. I am also assuming that the techniques are performed on a massage table.

Sternocleidomastoid

As most headaches are caused by the SCM, it is important to learn these techniques thoroughly. Almost all of my headache patients suffer from this.

Pressing Straight Into Neck

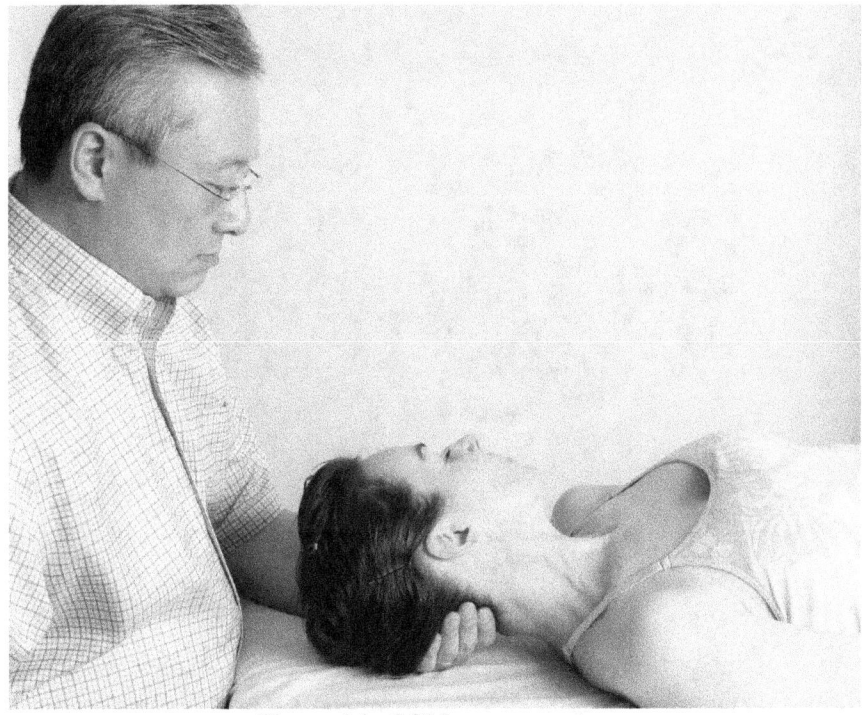

Figure 4.1 - SCM massage setup

Have the patient lie down facing up on a massage table. Sit behind the patient's head. Adjust the chair so that your forearms are comfortably resting on the massage table. If you can rest your feet flat comfortably on the floor, that is even better. The more comfortable you are, the better you can pay attention to the patient.

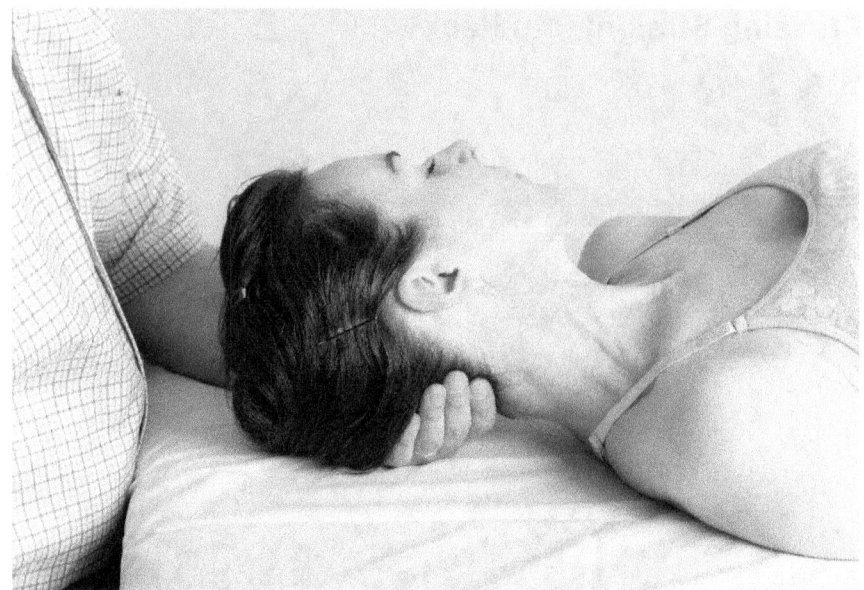

Figure 4.2 - SCM massage left hand setup

To treat the right SCM, place the left hand on the table, palm side up, and have the patient rest the head on the palm. The pad of the left thumb is placed on the left mastoid process of the head, and the pads of the third and fourth fingers on the right mastoid process. This is so that you can control the position of the head and neck easily while the patient lies passively on the table. Rest the second and fifth fingers wherever they land naturally.

Rotate the head to the left about 45 degrees. Visibly locate the SCM. The muscle has two heads. They are both attached to the mastoid process superiorly, and one head attaches to the sternum and the other attaches to the clavicle. Once located, put the pad of your right thumb on top of the muscle right below the mastoid process. While gently pressing on the muscle, slightly rotate the head left and right to find the optimum rotation where the muscle is taught enough to respond to the pressure, but not too tight so that it starts to contract. If the muscle is too loose, the pressure will simply go straight through the muscle to the underlying tissues instead. If the muscle is too tight, it causes additional and unnecessary pain during the treatment. The optimum angle of rotation will change as the muscles release, so you will need to constantly adjust throughout the session.

This is a skill that develops over time. Once the optimum angle is found, hold the head with the left hand to stabilize it by squeezing the thumb against the fingers. The patient should feel as though the head is being securely cradled in your hand.

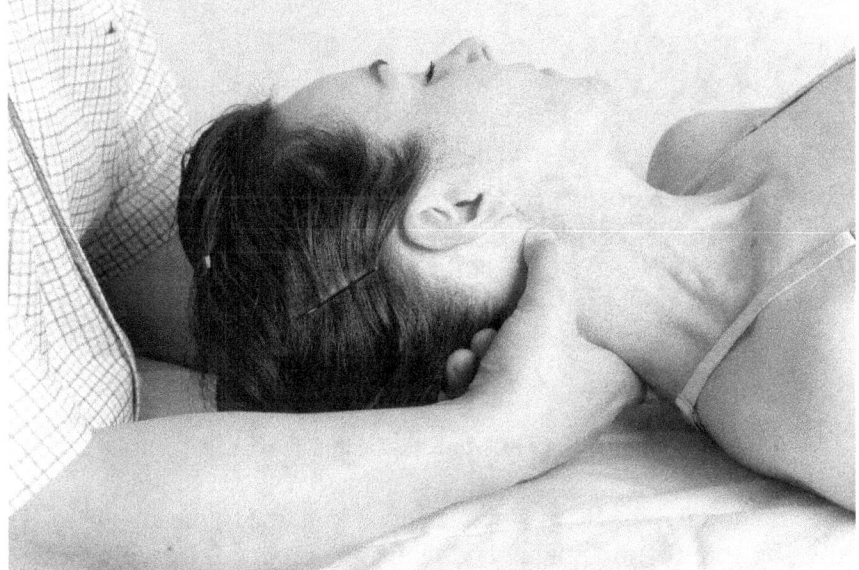

Figure 4.3 - SCM press straight into neck

Once the setup is complete, gradually press the right thumb perpendicularly into the SCM toward the center of the neck. Determining the correct amount of pressure is the hardest part of all the techniques in this book. If it is too light, then the muscles have no reasons to respond. On the other hand, if it is too heavy, then the muscle contracts further to protect itself. The best instruction I can give is to gradually increase the pressure until you "match" the pressure the muscle gives back to you. Once you feel the fasciculation under the thumb, although it can happen elsewhere in the neck, then you have passed the most difficult part in mastering the techniques. For the remainder of the treatment session, you will constantly look for ways to induce the fasciculation even more by varying rotation of the neck, pressure and direction of the thumb.

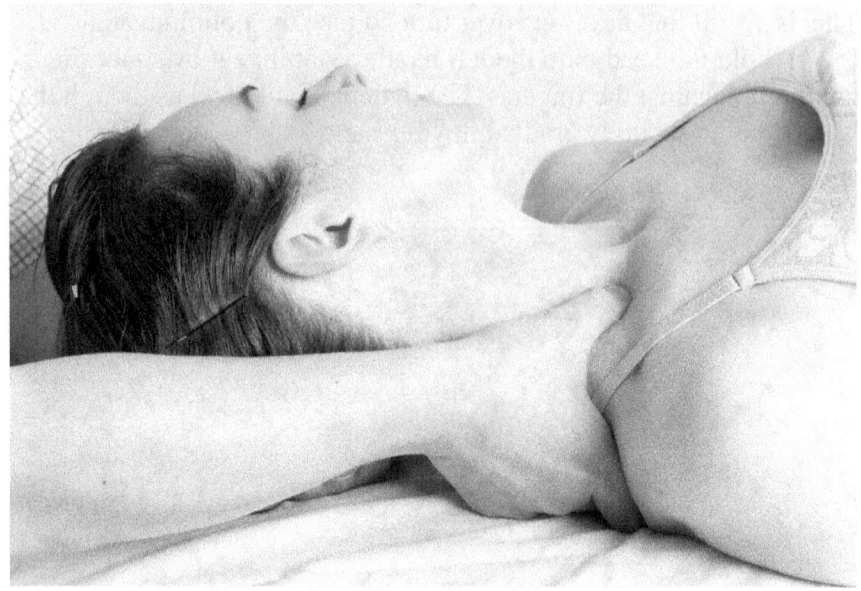
Figure 4.4 - SCM press straight into neck

Once the top part of SCM stops fasciculating, move the right hand down by about ½ of an inch, and repeat the process. Continue this process until you have finished both heads of the muscle. For some patients, the heads split quite apart from each other near the bottom attachments. In this case, you will have to treat each head separately. For most patients, they are close enough together, in which case, you aim for the bulky middle part.

As you move down along the muscle, the patient will surely say something like "ah, you are recreating the same headache I've been having." Stay there longer even after the fasciculation stops until the patient tells you that the elicited headache has more or less disappeared, or the reduction in the headache hits a plateau. If the headache disappears completely, great, keep moving down along the muscle. If you reach a plateau, that is okay. You will get it with the subsequent techniques.

Pressing Up to Detach

The purpose of this technique and the next is to free the SCM from its surrounding tissues. The tension of the muscle is not only within itself, but can come from its inability to move or glide freely away from the surrounding tissues. This and the following techniques solve this issue.

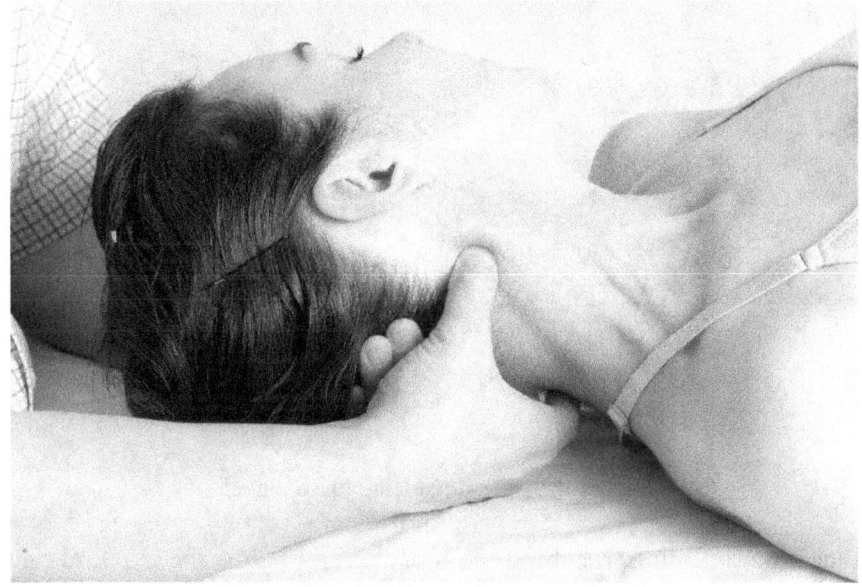

Figure 4.5 - SCM pressing up to detach

The setup of this technique is identical to the previous technique. The difference between this technique and the previous one is that instead of pressing the thumb perpendicularly toward the center of the neck, the thumb is placed posterior to the muscle so that it can push the muscle away anteriorly from the posterior tissues.

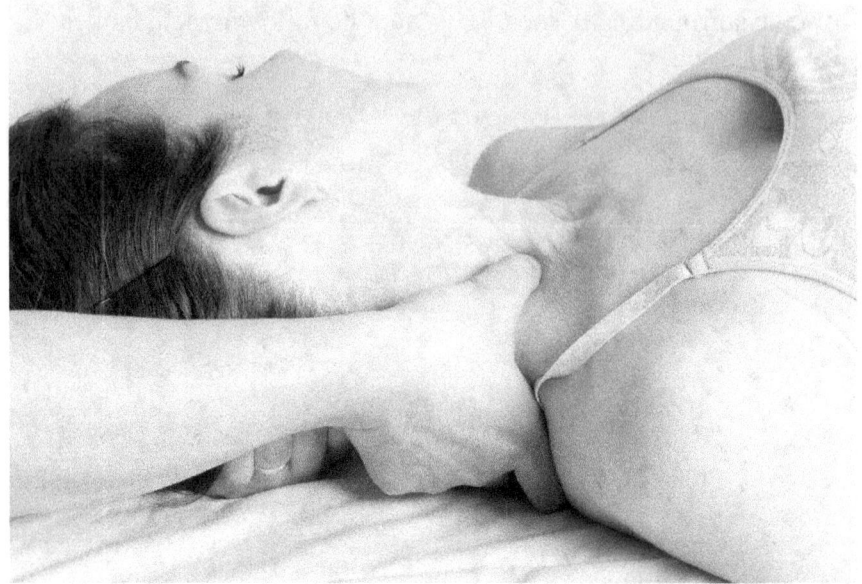
Figure 4.6 - SCM pressing up to detach

Place the right thumb behind the muscle right below the mastoid process, and slightly press perpendicularly into the center of the neck to be able to get behind the muscle fiber first, and then press anteriorly to push the muscle away from the table toward the ceiling. Just like the previous technique, the muscle will fasciculate. Repeat this process ½ inch by ½ inch.

Pressing Down to Detach

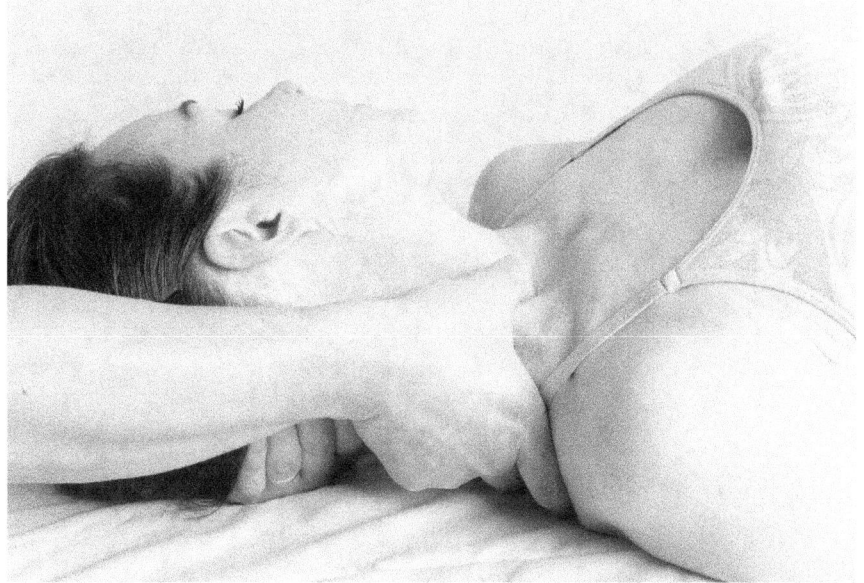

Figure 4.7 - SCM pressing down to detach

This technique is identical to the second technique except the direction of the pressure is posterior toward the table to detach the muscle from the anterior tissues.

Squeeze the Rest

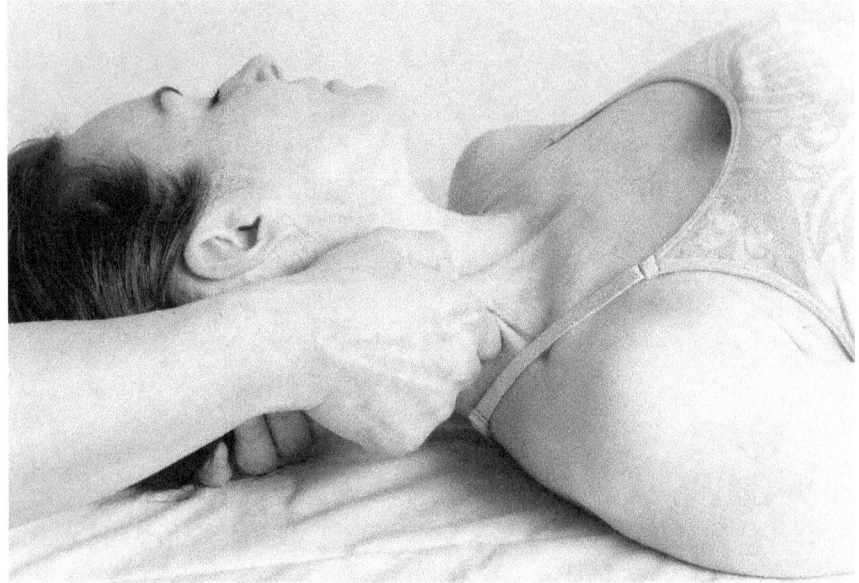

Figure 4.8 - SCM squeeze the rest

I used to use this technique only for many years before incorporating the first three techniques. It is that important and potent. But, I perform this after the three pressing techniques as they reduce the pain felt by the patient substantially.

This technique is rather simple. You squeeze the muscle between the thumb and the index finger from the top to bottom. Various parts will cause headaches at different places. You hold until the elicited headaches disappear, and then move on. You may need to repeat this technique a couple of times to get rid of the remaining headaches.

The techniques for releasing the SCM are the hardest to learn. The rest of the techniques are substantially easier.

Temporalis

Before treating the temporalis, be sure to treat the SCM first. Temporalis is an extension of the SCM as far as headaches are concerned.

Have the patient lie down facing up on a massage table. Sit behind the patient's head. Adjust the chair so that your forearms are comfortably resting on the massage table. If you can rest your feet flat comfortably on the floor, that is even better. The more comfortable you are, the better you can pay attention to the patient.

Cover the left temporalis of the patient with the palm of your left hand to stabilize the head. You are not pushing the head to the right with the left palm. You are simply providing stability against the pushing that will come from the right thumb pressing into the head.

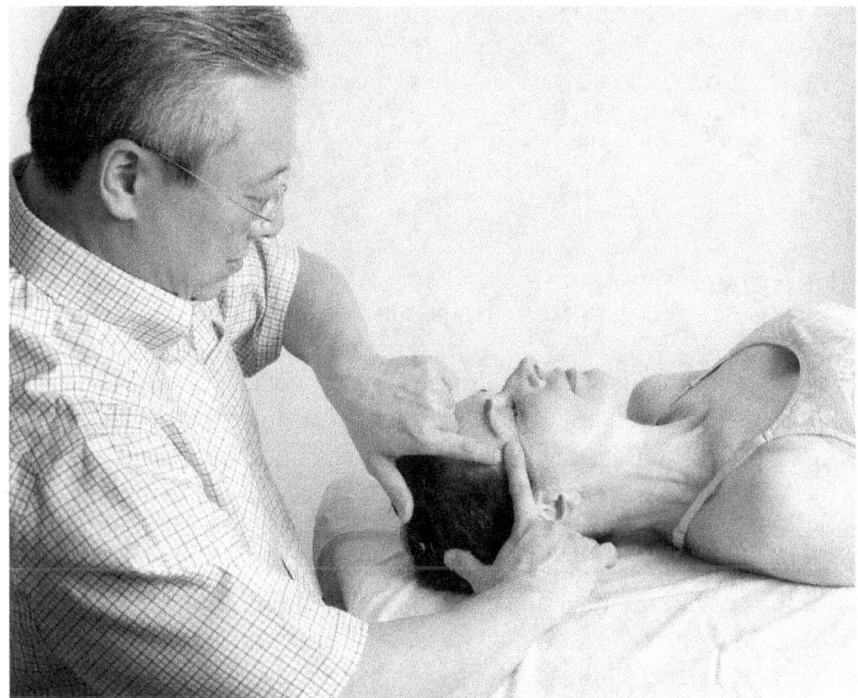

Figure 4.9 – Temporalis location

Once the setup is complete, gently place the middle three fingers on the right temporal area, and ask the patient to clench the jaw a few times. You will feel the temporalis jump against the fingers with each clench as it is a chewing muscle. Unlike the SCM, not all the muscle fibers need to be massaged. The lower fibers, which are about one finger width above the zygomatic arch, are all that are involved with headaches. Unlike the SCM techniques, which create unpleasant pain, the patients usually rather enjoy the firm massage of the temporalis.

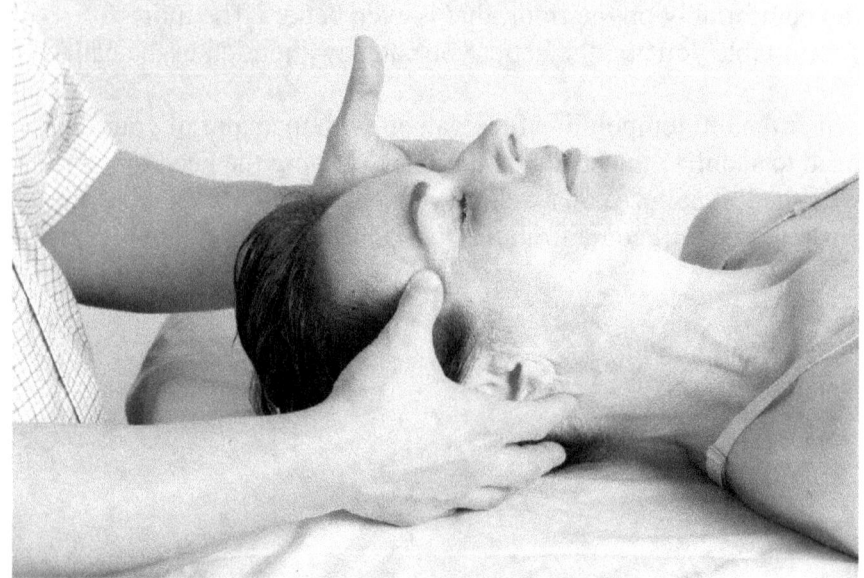

Figure 4.10 – Temporalis anterior fibers

Press the temporalis with the thumb starting near the eye. Ask the patient again to clench to make sure that your thumb is still on the temporalis. Unlike the SCM, fasciculation is not very obvious in the temporalis, so it is better to rely on the changes in the firmness of the muscle. The muscle will feel like a piece of dried chewing gum. Within 30 seconds or so, it will start to soften. Keep the pressure on until the softening hits a plateau. Move the thumb toward the ear by ¼ of an inch, and repeat the process until you reach the ear. If the patient experiences a headache from the pressure, hold the pressure until the headache disappears.

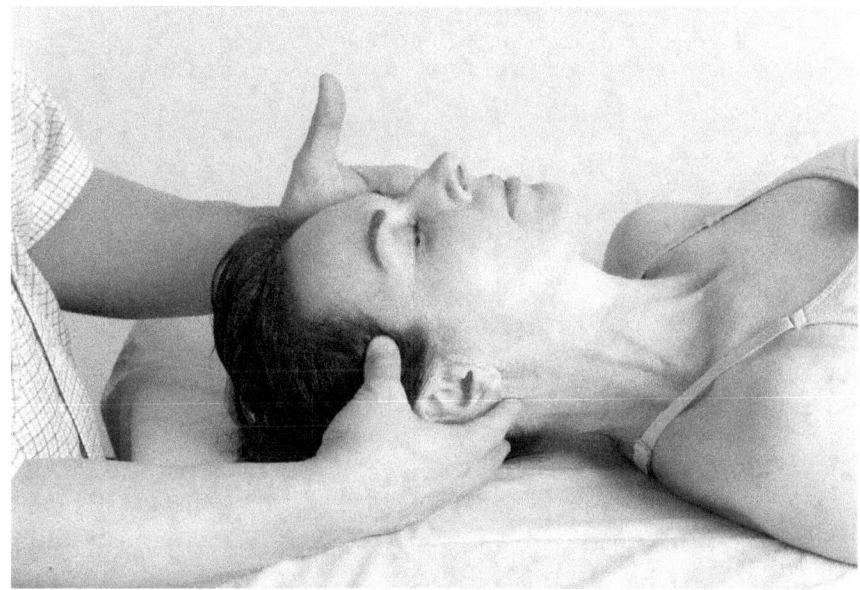

Figure 4.11 – Temporalis posterior fibers

Scalenes

As discussed, the scalenes need to be treated before treating either levator scapula or trapezius.

Have the patient lie down facing up on a massage table. Sit on the right side of the patient's head. Adjust the chair so that your left forearm is comfortably resting on the massage table. If you can rest your feet flat comfortably on the floor, that is even better. The more comfortable you are, the better you can pay attention to the patient.

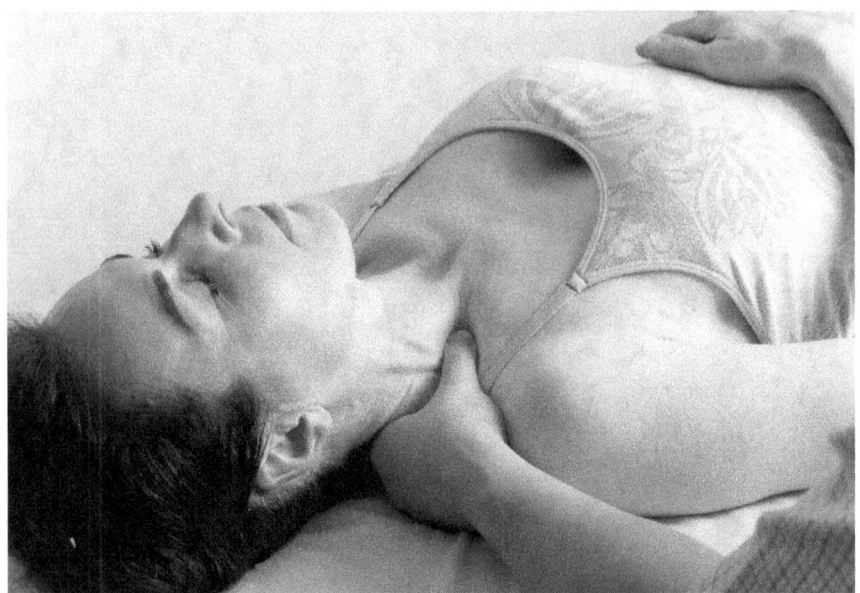
Figure 4.12 – Scalenes lower fibers

Stabilize the patient's neck by placing the four fingers of the left hand behind the nape of the neck. Put the pad of the left thumb lateral to the clavicular insertion of the SCM to contact the medial heads of the scalene. If the patient is thin and your palpatory skills are advanced enough to discern the anterior and medial heads of the muscle, you can massage them individually, but it is not necessary. Start with the inferior fibers, and work your way up to the superior fibers.

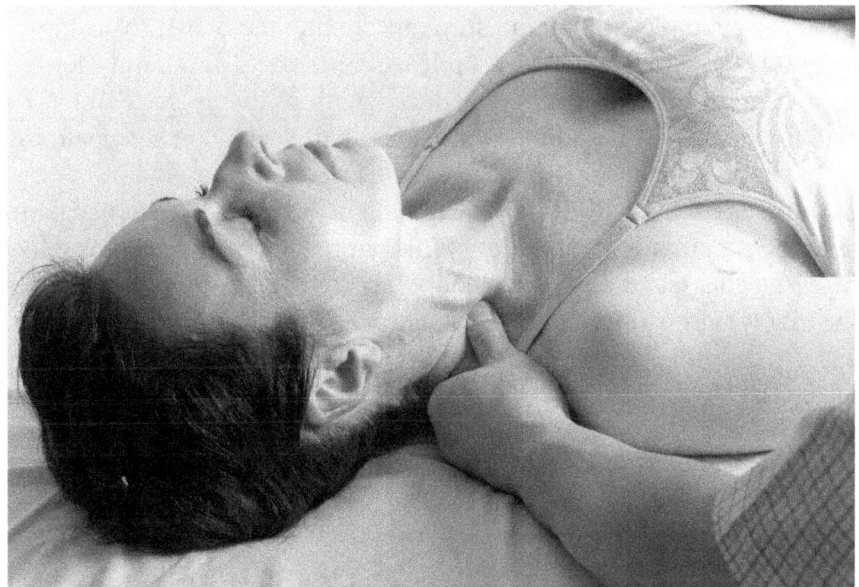
Figure 4.13 – Scalenes middle fibers

The fasciculation of these muscles is always overshadowed by the much bigger fasciculation of the levator scapula and upper trapezius, so instead of focusing on the thumb, focus on the fingers which are placed on the levator scapula and trapezius near the nape of the neck. The fasciculation is typically large enough for the patient to feel as well. When the fasciculation quiets down, move the thumb ¼ of an inch superior, and repeat the process. For an average size adult, 1.5 inch of thorough massage is enough to cover the belly of the muscles. There is no need to go higher than that.

The posterior head of scalenes does not seem to influence the levator scapula and trapezius much, so there is no need to massage this part of the muscle for headaches.

Levator Scapula

Levator scapula is better known for causing neck pain along the postolateral region of the neck down to the superior angle of the scapula that makes it hard to rotate the head to the contralateral side. As far as the headache goes, it causes headaches near the bottom of occiput just like the trapezius.

Levator scapula is a long and slim muscle like the SCM; releasing one part of the muscle does not release other parts of the muscle, making it necessary to treat the entire length of the muscle. What I find interesting is that the tension in one part seems to cause pain in other parts of the muscle instead of where the tension is. For example, patients with levator scapula tension often experience pain near the scapular insertion area. This part of the muscle can usually be easily massaged out with a double thumb technique or the tip of the elbow with straight perpendicular pressure. However, there are cases where this pain comes from the upper parts along the neck instead.

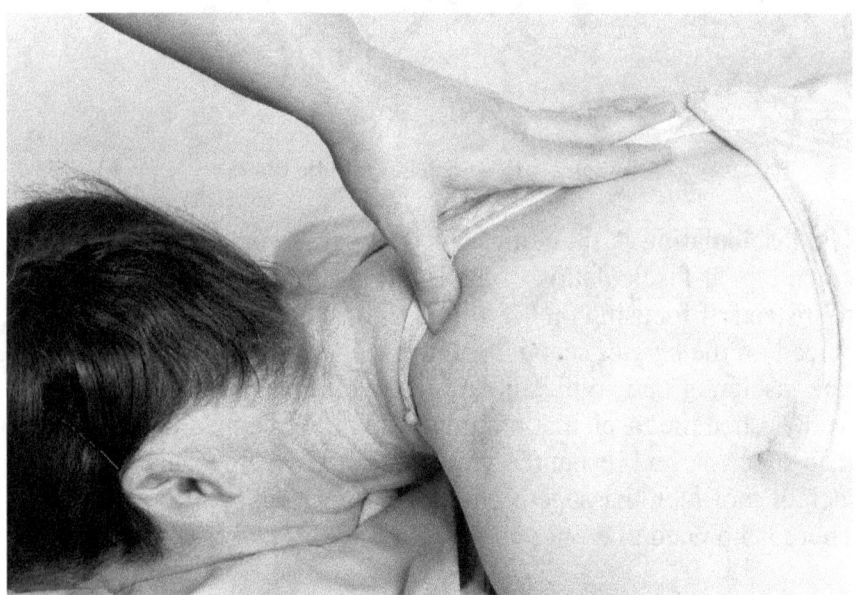

Figure 4.14 – Levator scapula scapular attachment (one thumb technique)

Start with the scapular insertion part of the muscle. Have the patient lie down facing down on a massage table. Stand behind the patient's head a little toward the patient's right shoulder. Depending on your strength and the size of the patient, use the thumb of the dominant hand, two thumbs on top of each other, or the tip of the elbow, and press perpendicularly into the body. Wait for the fasciculation to happen. The treatment of this part is complete when the fasciculation slows down to a complete stop.

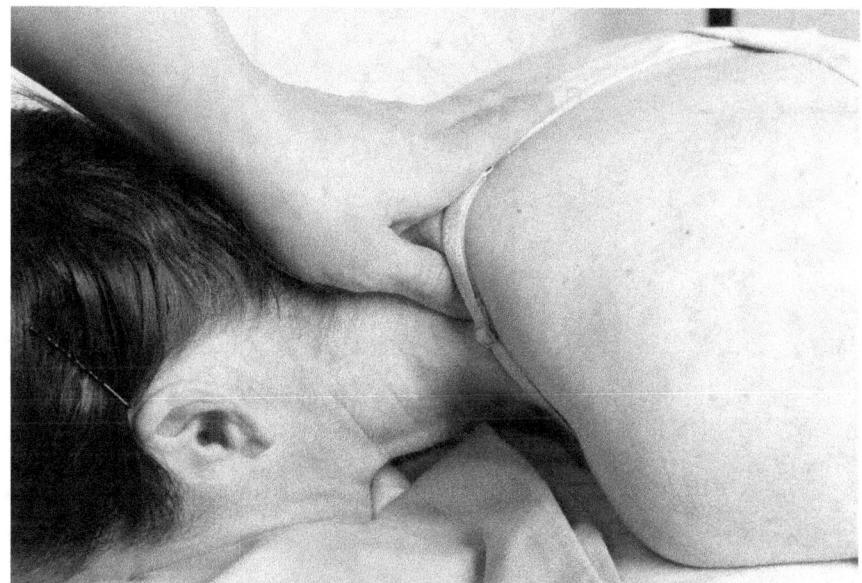
Figure 4.15 – Levator scapula nape of neck

The next part of the muscle to treat is at the nape of the neck. This part is partially covered by the trapezius. You need to go under the trapezius, find the levator scapula, and apply either the one thumb or the double thumb technique. The elbow is too big for this region. Wait for the fasciculation to happen. The treatment of this part is complete when the fasciculation slows down to a complete stop.

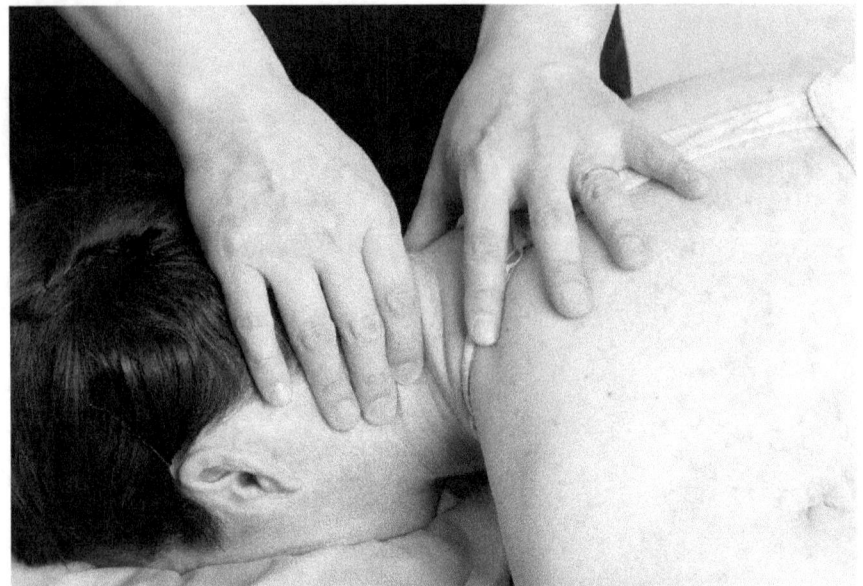

Figure 4.16 – Left levator scapula along neck

The remaining part of the muscle is along the neck. Move slightly to the patient's head toward the right shoulder so that you are facing the neck more so than the first two techniques. Place the fingers on the left side of the neck to stabilize the neck. You are not to press the fingers into the neck. The fingers are placed there to support the neck against the thumb that will do the pressing.

Before placing the thumb, find the trapezius first which is located posterior to the levator scapula, and find the SCM which is located anterior to the levator scapula. The levator scapula is a thin muscle that lies between these two larger muscles. The muscle size near this area is about the diameter of a pencil. Once you find this muscle, place your thumb and press toward the center of the neck against the fingers on the other side. Releasing this area will release chronic pain in the scapular attachment area. Wait for the fasciculation to happen. The treatment of this part is complete when the fasciculation slows down to a complete stop. Repeat this process along the entire length of the muscle with a ½ inch increment toward the head.

Trapezius

The trapezius is a flat and yet very wide muscle that spans all the way from the posterior neck and shoulders down to the bottom of thoracic spine. Only the upper fibers contribute to headaches in the temporal and occipital areas.

The temporal headache from the trapezius is slightly posterior to the referral headache from the SCM or temporalis, and is caused by the tension in the belly of the muscles lying superior to the scapula. Although acupuncturists often needle GB21 to release the tension in this area, I do not find that this one small region causes headaches. Rather, the whole bulk of the muscle seems to participate in causing the headache in the temporal area. This might be because the temporal headache is not caused by a nerve pinched somewhere by trapezius, or a single trigger point embedded in the muscles, but rather by the pure biomechanical pull of the muscle to the side of the head. For this reason, the whole muscle belly needs to be thoroughly massaged. Since the trapezius is a large muscle, and is often overworked from stress which causes the shoulders to hike upward, you will have plenty of muscle knots to choose from, and you will not be able to release the whole muscles within one session.

It does not matter whether you start the massage from near the neck and work your way toward the shoulder or the other way around. I personally start from belly of the muscles, but this is nothing more than a habit.

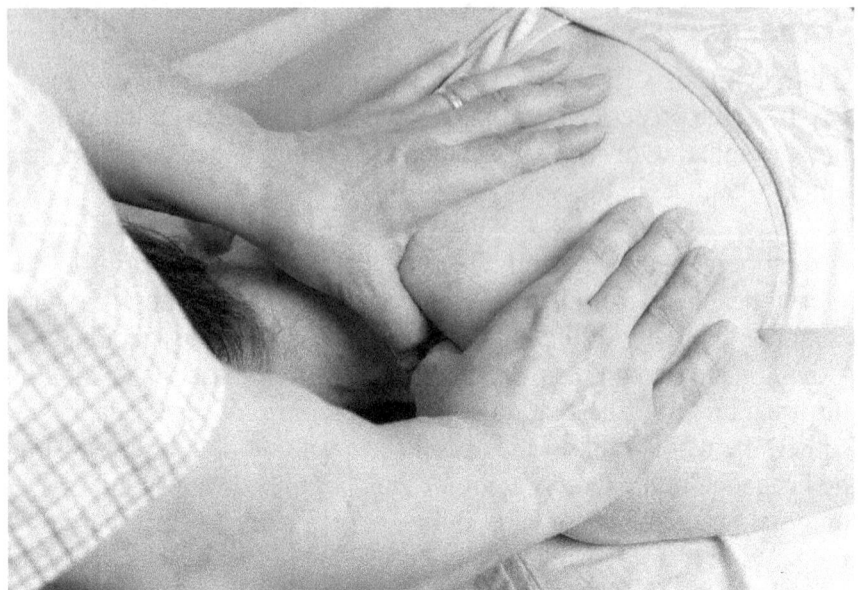
Figure 4.17 – Belly of trapezius

Place your thumbs side by side on top of the thickest portion of the muscle belly, and brace the hands by putting the fingers wherever they feel most comfortable. Gradually press the thumbs perpendicularly into the center of the muscle mass toward the feet. Of all the techniques in this book, you will use the most strength with the trapezius due to its sheer bulk. Remember that you are to "match" the pressure the muscle gives back to you, and the upper trapezius is big enough that you will the most likely need to press with your bodyweight behind the thumbs to find this match. The good thing about massaging this big muscle is that the fasciculation is big as well. Once the fasciculation stops, move along toward the shoulder by 1 inch, and repeat the process. Make sure not to press into the superior angle of the scapula. It's a bony projection, and hurts on everyone.

The occipital headache from the trapezius is slightly medial to the headache caused by levator scapula, and is caused by the tendinous part of the muscle at the exact attachment site on the occiput.

To treat the part of the trapezius that causes an occipital headache, we need to reposition the patient. The occipital attachment is not an easy place to release with pressure while the patient is lying face down, as the patient's face will be pressed against the face cradle or the hands if lying down on a bed. So, have the patient lie down facing up on a massage table. Sit behind the patient's head. Adjust the chair so that your forearms are comfortably resting on the massage table. If you can rest your feet flat comfortably on the floor, that is even better. The more comfortable you are, the better you can pay attention to the patient.

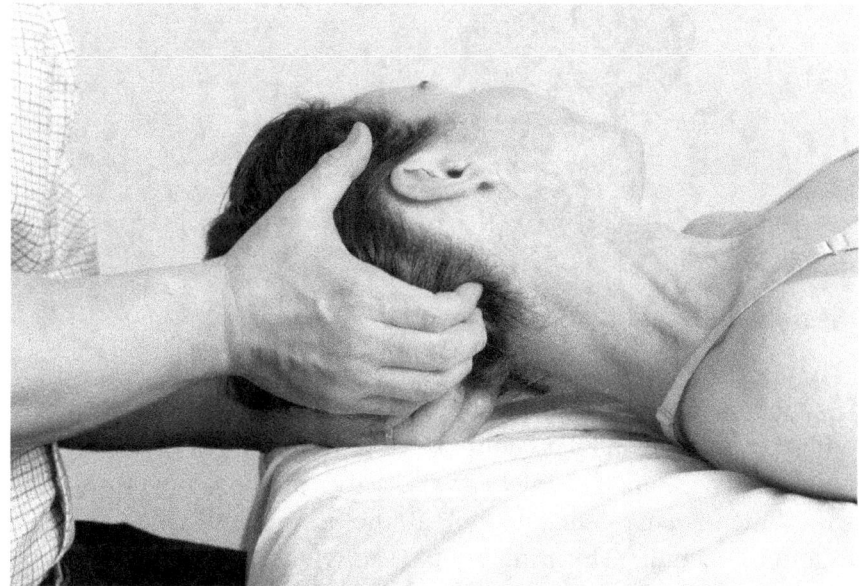

Figure 4.18 – Trapezius occipital attachment finger placement

Erect the middle 3 fingers of both hands so that the finger tips (not pads) are contacting the very bottom of the occiput, and move them up toward the vertex of the head by about 1.5 inches. This is the tendinous attachment site called external occipital protuberance. It is a little bumpy part on the occiput. It is not necessary to find this exact spot. Placing the fingers anywhere near is sufficient. What is necessary is to position the patient's head in your palms in such a way that the patient feels cradled so that the neck muscles can relax. You are to support all the weight of the head in your hands. If not, the patient will contract the neck muscles to lift the head, in which case it will be impossible for them to release. I often ask my patient to push the head against my palms, and then let go. This helps the patient to stop lifting the head.

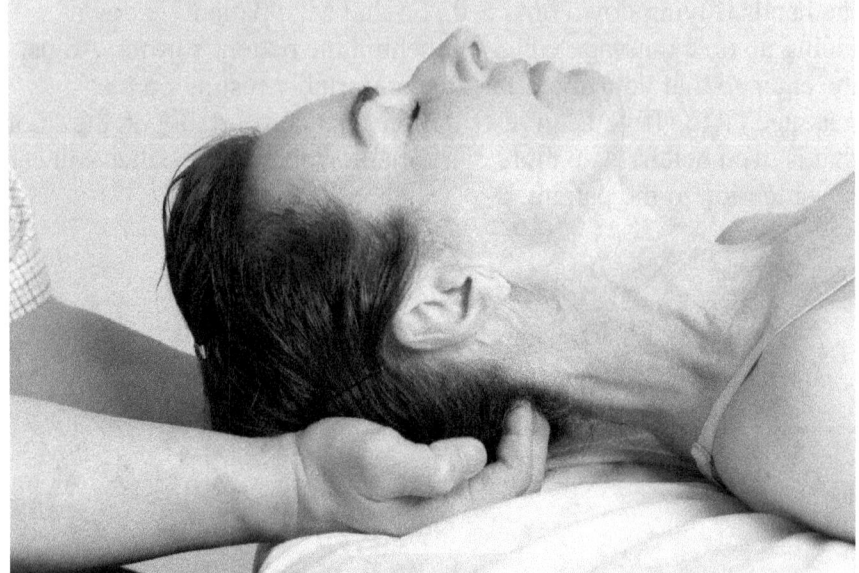

Figure 4.19 – Trapezius occipital attachment

The tendons will initially feel like a piece of dried out chewing gum. With the constant and yet gentle pressure from the gravity, they will slowly thaw and melt. Slowly and heavily drag your fingertips toward the patient's feet, and melt all the tissues until you get to the bottom of occiput. This is a very pleasurable technique for the patient, but can be hard on untrained fingers.

There are tools that do an excellent job at this; the DaVinci tool and the Real Ease. Start with the Real Ease as this tool is much safer than the DaVinci tool. The DaVinci tool, however, goes in much deeper, and is a better choice if the tissues are so hardened and thick from many decades of handling undue tension. Both of these tools can be purchased at Amazon.com. Follow the accompanying directions.

Masseter

Sinus infection and pressure intrigue me. I had thought that these were immune responses to pathogens such as viruses that cause the common cold. It turns out that that is not entirely correct. I have treated enough patients with sinus problems from a cold, and I can usually release the pressure within minutes, and the fluid starts to drain during the treatment, especially if the patients are in the early or later stages of the common cold. If the sinus problems are immune responses, how can they go away so fast? I wondered.

I eventually learned that acute sinus problems are caused by tension in the masseter, and the chronic or episodic problems by torsion in the maxilla. Treating bones like the maxilla is beyond the scope of this book, but massaging the masseter will still help with the chronic sinus problems, and eliminate acute sinus problems.

The masseter has two layers. They both attach to the angle of the jaw bone, but the deep one goes to the posterior part of the zygomatic arch toward the temple whereas the superficial one goes to the anterior part of the zygomatic arch toward the eye. It is the superficial layer that causes sinus problems whether the problems are pressure or infection.

Have the patient lie down facing up on a massage table. Sit behind the patient's head. Adjust the chair so that your forearms are comfortably resting on the massage table. If you can rest your feet flat comfortably on the floor, that is even better. The more comfortable you are, the better you can pay attention to the patient.

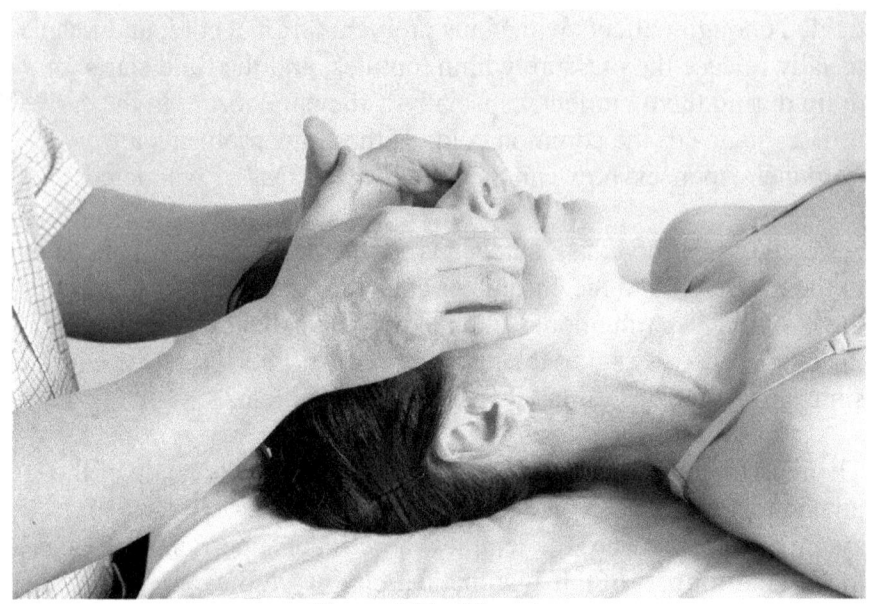
Figure 4.20 – Masseter

Place the tips of the middle 3 fingers on the face right below the zygoma, and make gentle contact with the maxilla. And, stay there. Unlike the other techniques that depended on brute force, this technique is more about getting the muscle tissues engaged. Close your eyes, quiet your mind, and concentrate on the tiny movements of the muscle tissues at your fingertips.

You will not feel an obvious fasciculation, but the patient will feel the pressure and congestion slowly but surely disappear. During that time, you may feel some tissue anomalies that feel like rice grains (something that is different from the surrounding tissues) under the finger tips disappear. Slightly move the finger tips around until you find more rice grains, and repeat the process. If you do not feel them, that is okay. The disappearance of the pressure and congestion perceived by the patient is much more important and reliable feedback. When this technique is performed correctly, the whole treatment should take less than ten minutes.

Chapter 5 – Perpetuating Factors

If the muscle tension causes headaches, then what causes muscle tension in the first place? This is a very hard question to answer, and is worthy of multiple PhD theses, exploring not only physiological aspects, but also emotional and even spiritual aspects, which is beyond my expertise. I will discuss some of these that I commonly see in my practice. Hopefully, the readers will find one or more that make you go "aha!" in which case eliminating them from your daily habits can put the headaches to rest for good.

Orthopedic Factors

Sleeping Posture

The most common daily habit that I see among headache sufferers is bad sleeping postures that put the neck and head in positions that make the 6 muscles chronically tense.

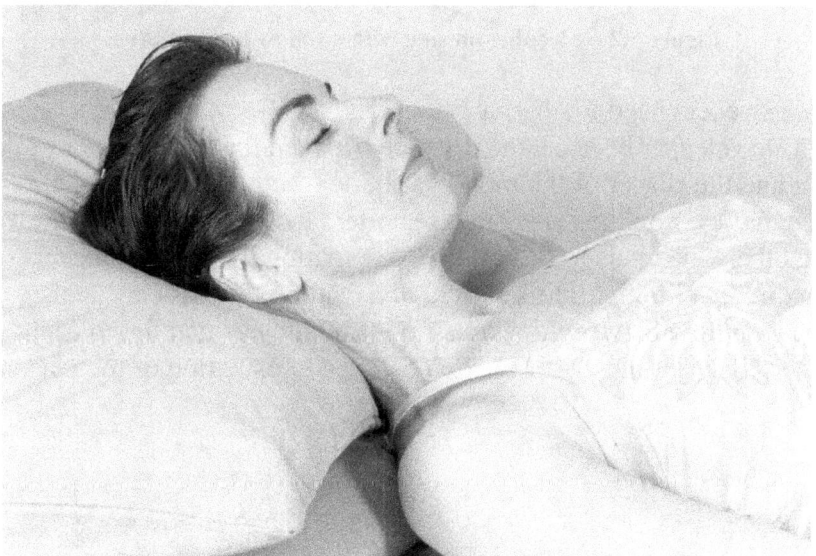

Figure 5.1 – Sleeping on back with multiple pillows

Back sleepers typically use multiple pillows or down pillows that put the head and neck in a forward position all night long, resulting in shortened SCM and scalenes, and lengthened trapezius and levator scapula. Lengthening a muscle under load causes muscle knots, and shortening a muscle causes the surrounding fascia to tighten over an extended period of time, both of which can cause headaches.

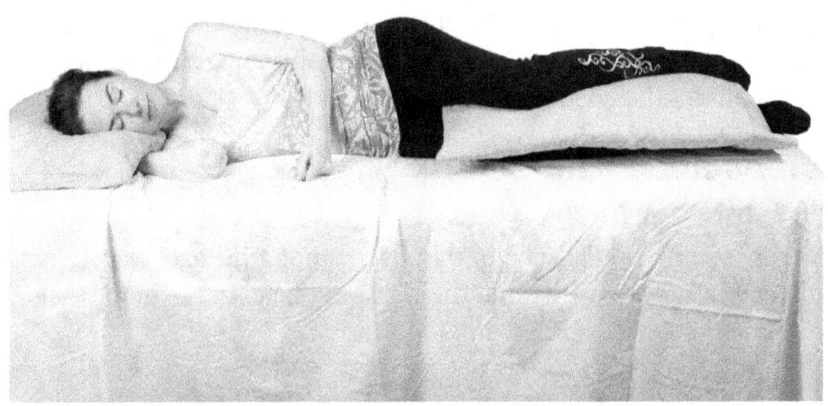

Figure 5.2 – Sleeping on side with a pillow between knees

Side sleepers need to alternate the sides. I can always tell if a patient is a side sleeper because the distance between the outer corner of the eye and the corner of the mouth is shorter on the side that is slept on. The masseter on the same side is shorter, and the joint of the jaw on the other side tends to be painful. Alternating the side whenever waking up eliminates this structural deviation. Side sleepers also need a pillow between the knees to make the legs parallel to each other. See "sitting posture" for a detailed explanation of the reasons.

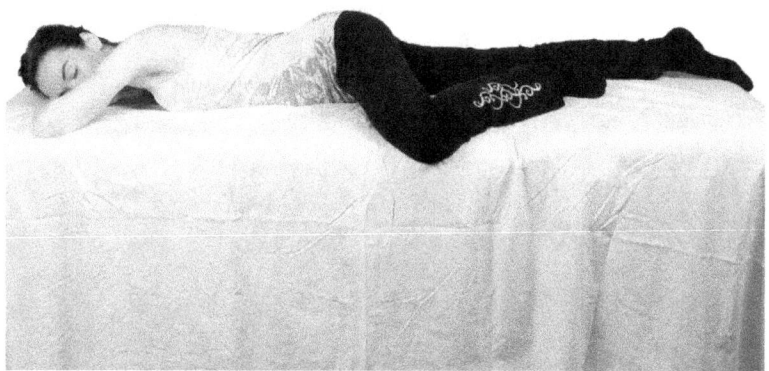

Figure 5.3 – Sleeping on stomach

Stomach sleepers basically need to stop sleeping on the stomach. This sleeping posture severely rotates not only the neck, but the entire torso. There is no cure in the world that can undo what stomach sleeping does for hours every night.

Recommending the right pillow is very hard as individual needs are as varied as fingerprints. What I would recommend is to have someone look at you on the pillow to make sure that the head and the torso are aligned. If the pillow has the right contour and thickness, the head will not tilt forward or backward, be pushed forward, or pulled backward. It will take at least a couple of weeks to get comfortable with a new pillow, so do not go by how comfortable the pillow feels when trying out a new pillow. An easy way to determine the correct thickness is to use a bathroom towel. Fold it in layers until you find the thickness that satisfies my guidelines. That is what I do when I travel and sleep in hotels as most hotel pillows are way too thick for me. Remember that pillows are there to support your neck, not your head.

Sitting Posture

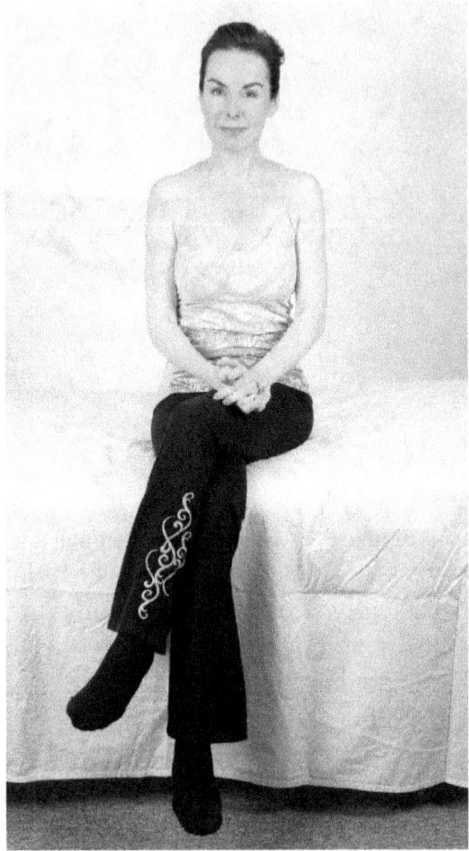
Figure 5.4 – Sitting with legs crossed

Crossing one leg over the other typically anteriorly rotates the pelvis, making the leg functionally longer than the other. Sleeping on one side where the legs are not parallel to each other, or the top leg rests in front of the bottom leg creates an identical problem, hence the suggestion of putting a pillow between the knees. This uneven hip creates asymmetrical bending and torsion along the spine and neck, creating unnatural constant mechanical loading in the neck muscles, which then create a headache. Just like side sleeping, alternate the legs if you have to cross your legs when sitting. Better yet, do not cross your legs at all.

Breathing

Breathing is so important in so many aspects of health that it deserves a tome all by itself. As far as the physiological aspect of the breathing in the narrow scope of headaches goes, the diaphragm needs to drive the inhalation of the air by moving downwards, not the neck muscles lifting the rib cage upward. While either mechanics will create negative pressure in the lungs so that the air will come in, the tiny neck muscles are simply not designed to lift the heavy ribs tens of thousands of times a day, and yet so many people, especially women, tend to breathe like this. The neck muscles naturally become fatigued, which then leads to trigger point development, which then creates headaches. You get the picture.

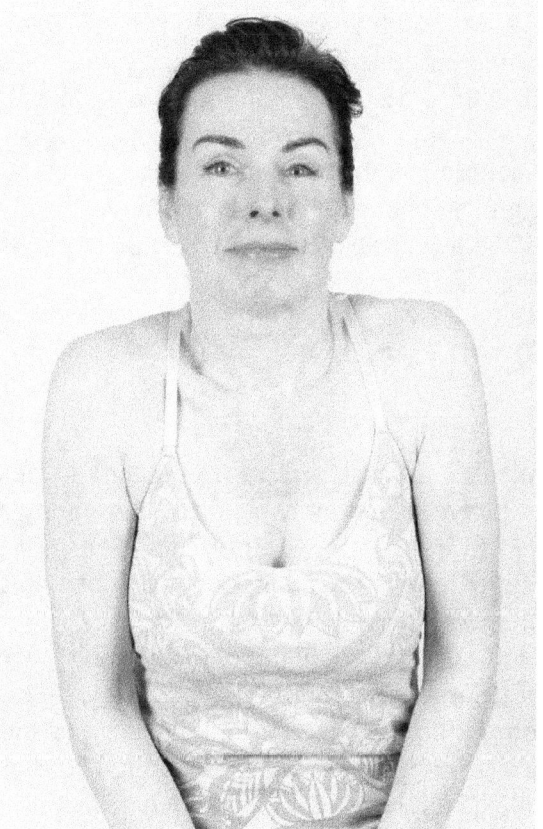

Figure 5.5 – Breathing by lifting chest

The constant up and down movement of the diaphragm gently massages the internal organs, including the large intestine. Most patients with chronic constipation simply do not have enough diaphragm movement. I suspect that the peristalsis of the large intestine is not powerful enough to move the feces along. The large intestine needs to be massaged by the diaphragm for optimum bowel movement. The chronic headache sufferers with constipation issues would be wise to check whether they breathe diaphragmatically.

Others

There are a lot of activities that can strain the neck muscles beyond what have been covered such as holding a baby on one side of the hip while the dominant hand is doing something else, having a TV or computer monitor off to one side, holding a telephone with a shoulder, etc. Go through your daily activities in your mind, and see if you do anything one sided for a prolonged period of time, and learn to alternate the sides or stop doing them all together.

One of my patients spent many hours talking on the phone wedged between his right ear and the shoulder. It was not until he stopped doing this that the headache went away permanently. He opted to use a speaker phone instead.

Internal Organ Factors

Liver

Almost all patients I have treated have a bigger and tenser SCM on the right side. I have seen only two exceptions among more than a thousand patients I have seen over the years. I suspect that this is because the bigger lobe of the liver is on the right side, making the right side of the torso heavier, forcing the right SCM take on more load than the left SCM. Although there is nothing that can be done about having the larger lobe on the right side, decongesting the liver can still be done by doing a liver & gallbladder flushing, and lightening the load on the right SCM. Although controversial, I have seen undeniable health benefits in my patients who have done this flushing. More information on the benefits and flushing procedure can be found on my website (https://healingbyyang.com/liver-and-gallblader-cleansing/).

Leaky Gut

There is a lot of information online about leaky gut. The summary is that fecal matters leak through the membranes of the small and large intestines into the bloodstream, causing health problems, one of them being headaches. If you have allergies, skin issues, or immune system issues, you may want to have this treated. My preference is using colostrum. Make sure that it is not processed with heat, which nullifies all the health benefits of colostrum.

Diet

All the headache books in the market seem to focus on dietary causes of headaches. The information is very thorough and I do not have much to add. If I were to summarize these books, it would come down to not eating anything that your great, great, grandmother would not recognize, such as a TV dinner, processed food, and GMOs. They are simply not food.

References

[1] Source obtained from the Internet:
http://headacheandmigrainenews.com/vasoconstrictor-migraine-headaches/
[2] Source obtained from the Internet: https://migraine.com/migraine-treatment/imitrex/
[3] Source obtained from the Internet:
http://headacheandmigrainenews.com/vasoconstrictor-migraine-headaches/
[4] Source obtained from the Internet:
https://www.scientificamerican.com/article/what-are-the-effects-of-a/
[5] Toussaint CP, Perry 3rd EC, Pisansky MT, Anderson DE. What's new in the diagnosis and treatment of peripheral nerve entrapment neuropathies. Neurol Clin. 2010;28(4):979-1004
[6] Andrea M. Trescot, Esther Warner, Matthew P. Rupert. Peripheral nerve entrapments. Clinical diagnosis and management. 2016;93
[7] Kopell HP, Thompson WA. Peripheral entrapment neuropathies. Baltimore: Williams and Wilkins; 1976
[8] Andrea M. Trescot, Rafael Justiz. Peripheral nerve entrapments. Clinical diagnosis and management. 2016;185-186
[9] Travell JG, Simons DG. Myofascial pain and dysfunction. The trigger point manual, the upper extremities. Vol 1. Baltimore: Williams & Wilkins; 1983;292
[10] Travell JG, Simons DG. Myofascial pain and dysfunction. The trigger point manual, the upper extremities. Vol 1. Baltimore: Williams & Wilkins; 1983;5-44
[11] Travell JG, Simons DG. Myofascial pain and dysfunction. The trigger point manual, the upper extremities. Vol 1. Baltimore: Williams & Wilkins; 1983;60-62
[12] Travell JG, Simons DG. Myofascial pain and dysfunction. The trigger point manual, the upper extremities. Vol 1. Baltimore: Williams & Wilkins; 1983;202-204
[13] Travell JG, Simons DG. Myofascial pain and dysfunction. The trigger point manual, the upper extremities. Vol 1. Baltimore: Williams & Wilkins; 1983;203-204
[14] Source obtained from the Internet:
https://www.ncbi.nlm.nih.gov/books/NBK11042/
[15] Travell JG, Simons DG. Myofascial pain and dysfunction. The trigger point manual, the upper extremities. Vol 1. Baltimore: Williams & Wilkins; 1983;240
[16] Travell JG, Simons DG. Myofascial pain and dysfunction. The trigger point manual, the upper extremities. Vol 1. Baltimore: Williams & Wilkins; 1983;240
[17] Travell JG, Simons DG. Myofascial pain and dysfunction. The trigger point manual, the upper extremities. Vol 1. Baltimore: Williams & Wilkins; 1983;336
[18] Travell JG, Simons DG. Myofascial pain and dysfunction. The trigger point manual, the upper extremities. Vol 1. Baltimore: Williams & Wilkins; 1983;334-335
[19] Travell JG, Simons DG. Myofascial pain and dysfunction. The trigger point manual, the upper extremities. Vol 1. Baltimore: Williams & Wilkins; 1983;185

[20] Andrea M. Trescot, Agnes R. Stogicza. Peripheral nerve entrapments. Clinical diagnosis and management. 2016;259

[21] Travell JG, Simons DG. Myofascial pain and dysfunction. The trigger point manual, the upper extremities. Vol 1. Baltimore: Williams & Wilkins; 1983;186

[22] Travell JG, Simons DG. Myofascial pain and dysfunction. The trigger point manual, the upper extremities. Vol 1. Baltimore: Williams & Wilkins; 1983;346

[23] Source obtained from the Internet: https://www.ncbi.nlm.nih.gov/books/NBK11042/

[24] Travell JG, Simons DG. Myofascial pain and dysfunction. The trigger point manual, the upper extremities. Vol 1. Baltimore: Williams & Wilkins; 1983;219-221

[25] Travell JG, Simons DG. Myofascial pain and dysfunction. The trigger point manual, the upper extremities. Vol 1. Baltimore: Williams & Wilkins; 1983;61

[26] Travell JG, Simons DG. Myofascial pain and dysfunction. The trigger point manual, the upper extremities. Vol 1. Baltimore: Williams & Wilkins; 1983;62